Soothe Your Soles

A Comprehensive Guide to Foot Care for Cracked Heels

Shahnaz Afroj Tuli

Table of Contents

Introduction

What is dry feet?

Dry feet refer to the condition in which the skin on the feet becomes excessively dry, rough, and cracked. This can occur when the skin on the feet loses its natural moisture and oil, leading to dryness and flakiness. Dry feet can be uncomfortable and unsightly, and can also lead to complications such as cracking and infection if left untreated. There are many factors that can contribute to dry feet, including genetics, age, climate, and lifestyle habits. Proper foot care, including regular moisturizing and exfoliation, can help prevent and treat dry feet.

What is cracked heels?

Cracked heels, also known as heel fissures, are a common foot condition characterized by dry, flaky skin on the heels that has become thickened and cracked. Cracked heels can be unsightly and uncomfortable, and in severe cases, they may cause pain or bleeding. The condition is often caused by a combination of factors, including dry skin, pressure on the feet, and medical conditions such as diabetes or psoriasis. Treatment for cracked heels typically involves regular moisturizing and exfoliation, as well as addressing any underlying medical conditions.

What is foot fungus?

Foot fungus, also known as athlete's foot, is a common fungal infection that affects the skin on the feet, particularly between the toes. It is caused by a group of fungi known as dermatophytes, which thrive in warm, moist environments like shoes and socks. Symptoms of foot fungus include redness, itching, scaling, and cracking of the skin on the feet. It can be treated with over-the-counter or prescription antifungal medications. Good foot hygiene, including keeping the feet clean and dry, wearing clean socks and shoes, and avoiding walking barefoot in public areas, can help prevent foot fungus.

Chapter 1: What Causes Cracked Heels?

Cracked heels are a common foot problem that can cause discomfort, pain, and even bleeding in severe cases. In this chapter, we will explore the various factors that can contribute to cracked heels, including dry skin, harsh soaps, medical conditions, and lifestyle habits. By understanding the root cause of cracked heels, readers can take steps to prevent future damage and maintain healthy feet.

Dry Skin:

One of the most common causes of cracked heels is dry skin. When the skin on the heels becomes dry, it can crack and split. This can be caused by a lack of moisture, hot and dry weather, or excessive bathing. In some cases, genetics may also play a role in the development of dry skin.

To prevent dry skin on the feet, it is important to keep them moisturized. Regularly applying a moisturizing cream or lotion can help to lock in moisture and prevent the skin from drying out. It is also important to avoid hot showers or baths, as these can further strip the skin of its natural oils. Instead, opt for lukewarm water and limit bathing time to 10-15 minutes.

Harsh Soaps and Detergents:

Using harsh soaps and detergents can also contribute to the development of cracked heels. These products can strip the skin of its natural oils, leaving it dry and prone to cracking. This is especially true for soaps and detergents that contain harsh chemicals or fragrances.

To prevent cracked heels caused by harsh soaps and detergents, it is important to choose gentle, mild products. Look for products that are specifically designed for sensitive skin, or opt for natural alternatives such as olive oil or coconut oil.

Medical Conditions:

Certain medical conditions can also contribute to the development of cracked heels. For example, diabetes can cause nerve damage and reduce circulation to the feet, making them more prone to dryness and cracking. Other medical conditions that can contribute to cracked heels include thyroid problems, psoriasis, and eczema.

If you suspect that an underlying medical condition may be contributing to your cracked heels, it is important to consult with a healthcare professional. They can help to diagnose and treat the condition, which can in turn help to improve the health of your feet.

Lifestyle Habits:

Certain lifestyle habits can also contribute to cracked heels. For example, standing for long periods of time can put pressure on the feet and cause them to become dry and cracked. Wearing ill-fitting shoes can also contribute to the development of cracked heels, as can neglecting foot care.

To prevent cracked heels caused by lifestyle habits, it is important to take care of your feet on a regular basis. This includes wearing supportive footwear, taking breaks to rest your feet if you stand for long periods of time, and practicing good foot hygiene. Regularly exfoliating the feet and moisturizing them can also help to prevent the development of cracked heels.

Cracked heels can be caused by a variety of factors, including dry skin, harsh soaps, medical conditions, and lifestyle habits. By identifying the root cause of their cracked heels, readers can take steps to prevent future damage and maintain healthy feet. This may include using moisturizing creams and lotions, wearing supportive footwear, and practicing good foot hygiene. In some cases, medical treatment may be necessary to address underlying health conditions that contribute to cracked heels.

Chapter 2: Preventing Cracked Heel

Preventing cracked heels is key to maintaining healthy feet. In this chapter, we will explore simple, daily habits that can help prevent cracked heels from developing in the first place. Topics include proper hydration, footwear choices, and foot care routines.

Proper Hydration:

One of the best ways to prevent cracked heels is to ensure that your body is properly hydrated. Drinking plenty of water throughout the day can help to keep the skin on your feet soft and supple. In addition to drinking water, eating a diet rich in fruits and vegetables can also help to keep your skin hydrated.

Footwear Choices:

Wearing the right footwear can also help to prevent cracked heels. Shoes that are too tight or too loose can put pressure on your feet, leading to dryness and cracking. To prevent this, it is important to choose shoes that fit properly and provide adequate support. Shoes made from breathable materials, such as leather or canvas, can also help to prevent moisture buildup that can lead to dry skin.

Foot Care Routines:

Regular foot care routines can also help to prevent cracked heels. This includes washing your feet daily with a mild soap and lukewarm water, and patting them dry with a soft towel. Applying a moisturizing cream or lotion to your feet after washing them can also help to lock in moisture and prevent dryness. It is also important to regularly exfoliate your feet to remove dead skin cells, which can contribute to the development of cracked heels.

Preventing cracked heels is a simple matter of incorporating healthy habits into your daily routine. By staying properly hydrated, choosing the right footwear, and maintaining a regular foot care routine, you can help to prevent dryness and cracking on your feet. Remember to consult with a healthcare professional if you experience persistent or severe symptoms, as this may be a sign of an underlying medical condition.

Chapter 3: Home Remedies for Cracked Heels

Cracked heels can be painful and uncomfortable, but there are several home remedies that can help to soothe and heal them. In this chapter, we will explore 10 effective home remedies for cracked heels.

Coconut Oil:

Coconut oil is a natural moisturizer that can help to soften and heal cracked heels. Simply apply a generous amount of coconut oil to your heels before bedtime and cover them with socks. Leave the socks on overnight and rinse your feet with lukewarm water in the morning.

Epsom Salt Soak:

Soaking your feet in a warm Epsom salt bath can help to soothe and heal cracked heels. Add one cup of Epsom salt to a tub of warm water and soak your feet for 15-20 minutes. Dry your feet thoroughly and apply a moisturizing cream or lotion.

Honey:

Honey has antibacterial and anti-inflammatory properties that can help to heal cracked heels. Mix one cup of honey with one cup of warm water and soak your feet in the mixture for 20 minutes. Rinse your feet with lukewarm water and pat them dry.

Oatmeal:

Oatmeal can help to soothe and moisturize dry, cracked heels. Mix one cup of oatmeal with warm water to create a paste. Apply the paste to your feet and let it sit for 30 minutes before rinsing it off with lukewarm water.

Lemon Juice:

Lemon juice has natural exfoliating properties that can help to remove dead skin cells from cracked heels. Mix equal parts lemon juice and warm water and soak your feet in the mixture for 20 minutes. Rinse your feet with lukewarm water and pat them dry.

Aloe Vera:

Aloe vera has anti-inflammatory properties that can help to soothe and heal cracked heels. Apply aloe vera gel directly to your heels and massage it into your skin. Leave it on for 15-20 minutes before rinsing it off with lukewarm water.

Vinegar:

Vinegar can help to exfoliate and soften dry, cracked heels. Mix one cup of vinegar with two cups of warm water and soak your feet in the mixture for 15-20 minutes. Rinse your feet with lukewarm water and pat them dry.

Petroleum Jelly:

Petroleum jelly can help to moisturize and protect cracked heels. Apply a generous amount of petroleum jelly to your heels before bedtime and cover them with socks. Leave the socks on overnight and rinse your feet with lukewarm water in the morning.

Banana:

Bananas are rich in vitamins and minerals that can help to heal cracked heels. Mash one ripe banana and apply the paste to your feet. Let it sit for 15-20 minutes before rinsing it off with lukewarm water.

Shea Butter:

Shea butter is a natural moisturizer that can help to soften and heal cracked heels. Apply a small amount of shea butter to your heels and massage it into your skin. Leave it on overnight and rinse your feet with lukewarm water in the morning.

Chapter 4: Medical Treatments for Cracked Heels

While many cases of cracked heels can be treated with home remedies and self-care, some may require medical intervention. In this chapter, we will explore the medical treatments available for cracked heels.

Prescription Creams:

If home remedies are not effective in treating cracked heels, a healthcare professional may recommend a prescription cream. These creams contain a higher concentration of active ingredients, such as urea, which can help to soften and heal dry, cracked skin.

Prescription creams are a common medical treatment for cracked heels that do not respond to home remedies. These creams contain higher concentrations of active ingredients, such as urea, which can help to soften and heal dry, cracked skin. Some commonly prescribed creams include:

Urea Cream:

Urea is a humectant that can attract and retain moisture in the skin, helping to soften and hydrate dry, cracked skin. Urea creams are available over-the-counter or by prescription, and may also contain other ingredients such as lactic acid, which can help to exfoliate dead skin cells.

Salicylic Acid Cream:

Salicylic acid is a keratolytic agent that can help to dissolve dead skin cells, making it a popular treatment for conditions such as psoriasis and warts. Salicylic acid creams are available over-the-counter or by prescription and may be used to treat cracked heels caused by thick, dry skin.

Steroid Cream:

In cases where cracked heels are caused by inflammation, a healthcare professional may prescribe a steroid cream. Steroid creams can help to reduce inflammation and promote healing of the skin. However, prolonged use of steroid creams can lead to skin thinning and other side effects, so it is important to use them as directed by a healthcare professional.

Laser Therapy:

Laser therapy is a relatively new treatment option for cracked heels. The procedure involves using a laser to heat and remove damaged tissue, which promotes the growth of healthy new skin. Laser therapy is generally considered safe and effective, but it can be costly and may require multiple sessions.

Laser therapy is a non-invasive medical treatment that can be used to promote the healing of cracked heels. During the procedure, a healthcare professional uses a laser to heat and remove damaged tissue from the affected area, which stimulates the growth of healthy new skin. The laser therapy can also help to reduce pain and inflammation associated with cracked heels.

Laser therapy is generally considered safe and effective, but it is not a one-time treatment and may require multiple sessions. The number of sessions required will depend on the severity of the cracked heels and the individual's response to treatment. Typically, treatments are spaced several weeks apart to allow the skin to heal in between sessions.

One of the main benefits of laser therapy is that it is a non-invasive procedure, meaning that it does not require any incisions or injections. This makes it a popular choice for individuals who may be hesitant to undergo more invasive medical treatments.

However, laser therapy can be costly and may not be covered by insurance. The cost of the procedure will depend on the healthcare provider and the specific type of laser used. It is important to discuss the potential cost and benefits of laser therapy with your healthcare provider before undergoing the procedure.

Footwear Modifications:

In some cases, cracked heels may be caused or exacerbated by footwear that does not fit properly. A healthcare professional may recommend modifications to your footwear, such as the use of orthotic inserts or wider shoes, to reduce pressure on the heels and promote healing.

Footwear modifications can be an effective treatment option for cracked heels that are caused or aggravated by ill-fitting shoes. A healthcare professional may recommend the following modifications to reduce pressure on the heels and promote healing:

Orthotic Inserts:

Orthotic inserts are specialized shoe inserts that can help to correct foot imbalances and reduce pressure on specific areas of the foot, such as the heels. These inserts can be custom-made by a healthcare professional or purchased over-the-counter.

Wider Shoes:

Wearing shoes that are too tight can cause increased pressure on the heels, leading to the development or worsening of cracked heels. Healthcare professionals may recommend wearing wider shoes or shoes with a larger toe box to reduce pressure on the foot and heel.

Cushioned Insoles:

Cushioned insoles can help to absorb shock and reduce pressure on the heels when walking or standing. These insoles can be purchased over-the-counter or prescribed by a healthcare professional.

It is important to follow the recommendations of your healthcare professional when modifying your footwear for cracked heels. Wearing improper footwear can worsen your symptoms and delay healing. If you have any questions or concerns about your footwear, consult with your healthcare professional.

Surgical Procedures:

In rare cases, surgery may be necessary to treat severe or persistent cases of cracked heels. A healthcare professional may recommend a procedure to remove damaged tissue, such as debridement, or to realign the bones in the foot to reduce pressure on the heels.

Surgical procedures are a last resort option for treating severe or persistent cases of cracked heels that have not responded to other treatments. Depending on the underlying cause of the cracked heels, a healthcare professional may recommend one of the following surgical procedures:

Debridement:

Debridement is a procedure that involves the removal of dead, damaged, or infected tissue from the affected area. In the case of cracked heels, debridement may involve removing the thick, callused skin that has formed around the heel to promote the growth of healthy new skin.

Bone Realignment:

If the cracked heels are caused by bone misalignment or other structural issues, a healthcare professional may recommend surgery to realign the bones in the foot. This can help to reduce pressure on the heels and prevent future episodes of cracked heels.

It is important to note that surgical procedures are typically reserved for severe or persistent cases of cracked heels and are not typically recommended as a first-line treatment option. Surgery can be expensive and may require a long recovery period, so it is important to discuss the potential risks and benefits of the procedure with your healthcare professional before making a decision.

Medical Conditions:

If cracked heels are caused by an underlying medical condition, such as diabetes or psoriasis, it is important to address the underlying condition in order to effectively treat the cracked heels. A healthcare professional can recommend appropriate treatments for the underlying condition, which may in turn help to heal the cracked heels.

Medical conditions can contribute to the development of cracked heels or make existing cracked heels more difficult to treat. If an underlying medical condition is identified as the cause of cracked heels, it is important to address the condition in order to effectively treat the cracked heels. Some common medical conditions that can contribute to cracked heels include:

Diabetes:

People with diabetes are at increased risk of developing cracked heels due to poor circulation and nerve damage. Diabetic foot care is important for preventing and treating cracked heels in people with diabetes.

Diabetes can cause damage to the nerves and blood vessels in the feet, which can lead to poor circulation and dry skin. Dry skin, in turn, can increase the risk of developing cracks and fissures in the heels. In severe cases, these cracks can become infected and lead to more serious foot problems, such as ulcers or even amputation.

To prevent and treat cracked heels in people with diabetes, it is important to practice good foot care. This includes:

- Regularly inspecting the feet for cracks, sores, or other signs of damage
- Keeping the feet clean and dry
- Moisturizing the feet regularly with a non-irritating moisturizer
- Avoiding harsh soaps and hot water
- Wearing well-fitting, comfortable shoes that do not rub or irritate the feet
- Avoiding going barefoot, even at home

Seeking medical attention promptly if any foot problems arise.

People with diabetes should also have regular foot exams by a healthcare professional to check for any signs of nerve damage or circulation problems. Good foot care can help prevent complications and keep the feet healthy and free from cracked heels.

Psoriasis:

Psoriasis is a chronic autoimmune condition that can cause thick, scaly patches of skin to form on the feet and elsewhere on the body. These patches can contribute to the development of cracked heels.

Psoriasis is a chronic autoimmune condition that affects the skin, causing it to become thick, scaly, and inflamed. Psoriasis can affect any part of the body, including the feet, and can cause dry, cracked skin on the heels and elsewhere.

Psoriasis can also cause joint pain and swelling, a condition called psoriatic arthritis. This can affect the feet and toes, causing pain, stiffness, and swelling that can contribute to the development of cracked heels.

To prevent and treat cracked heels in people with psoriasis, it is important to manage the underlying condition. This may include:

- Using topical treatments, such as corticosteroid creams or ointments, to reduce inflammation and soften thick, scaly skin
- Taking oral or injectable medications, such as biologics, to reduce inflammation and slow the progression of psoriasis
- Avoiding triggers that can exacerbate psoriasis symptoms, such as stress, certain medications, or skin injuries
- Moisturizing the feet regularly with a non-irritating moisturizer
- Wearing well-fitting, comfortable shoes that do not rub or irritate the feet
- Avoiding going barefoot, even at home

Seeking medical attention promptly if any foot problems arise.

Eczema:

Eczema is a common skin condition characterized by dry, itchy, and inflamed skin. People with eczema may be more prone to developing cracked heels due to the dryness and inflammation of the skin.

The dryness and inflammation can contribute to the development of cracked heels, particularly if the skin is not moisturized regularly.

To prevent and treat cracked heels in people with eczema, it is important to manage the underlying condition. This may include:

- Using topical treatments, such as corticosteroid creams or ointments, to reduce inflammation and soothe dry, itchy skin
- Applying moisturizer to the feet regularly, especially after bathing or swimming
- Avoiding triggers that can exacerbate eczema symptoms, such as harsh soaps, hot water, or stress
- Wearing soft, breathable shoes and socks
- Avoiding going barefoot, even at home
- Using gentle, fragrance-free products on the feet
- Seeking medical attention promptly if any foot problems arise.

Hypothyroidism:

Hypothyroidism is a condition in which the thyroid gland does not produce enough thyroid hormone. This can lead to dry skin, including on the feet and heels.

The thyroid hormone plays an important role in regulating skin health, so when levels are low, it can lead to dryness and other skin problems.

Regarding vitamin deficiencies, certain vitamins are essential for maintaining healthy skin, including vitamins A, C, and E. Deficiencies in these vitamins can lead to dry, rough, or scaly skin, which can contribute to the development of cracked heels.

To prevent and treat cracked heels due to vitamin deficiencies, it is important to ensure that you are getting enough of these vitamins in your diet or through supplements. Foods that are high in these vitamins include:

- Vitamin A: sweet potatoes, carrots, spinach, kale, and liver
- Vitamin C: citrus fruits, strawberries, broccoli, and bell peppers
- Vitamin E: almonds, sunflower seeds, and spinach
- Vitamin deficiencies can contribute to dry, cracked skin, including on the heels. Vitamins A and E, in particular, are essential for maintaining healthy skin. Vitamin A helps to promote cell growth and repair, while vitamin E is a powerful antioxidant that helps to protect skin cells from damage.

When there is a deficiency in these vitamins, the skin may become dry, rough, and prone to cracking. To prevent and treat cracked heels due to vitamin deficiencies, it is important to ensure that you are getting enough of these vitamins in your diet or through supplements.

Foods that are high in vitamin A include sweet potatoes, carrots, spinach, kale, and liver. Foods that are high in vitamin E include almonds, sunflower seeds, and spinach. Supplements may also be recommended by a healthcare professional if dietary sources are not enough.

Supplements may also be recommended by a healthcare professional if dietary sources are not enough.

While home remedies and self-care can be effective in treating many cases of cracked heels, some may require medical intervention. If you are experiencing persistent or severe symptoms, it is important to consult with a healthcare professional to determine the best course of treatment for your specific needs.

Chapter 5: Caring for Cracked Heels Long-Term

Here are some tips for maintaining healthy feet and preventing future episodes of cracked heels:

Daily Foot Care:

Develop a daily foot care routine that includes washing and drying your feet, moisturizing with a foot cream, and checking for any signs of skin damage or abnormalities. Keeping your feet clean and moisturized can help prevent dry skin and cracking.

- Wash your feet daily with warm water and a mild soap. Be sure to dry your feet thoroughly, especially between the toes, as excess moisture can contribute to fungal infections.

- Exfoliate your feet with a foot scrub or pumice stone to remove dead skin cells and promote circulation.

- Apply a moisturizing foot cream or lotion to your feet, focusing on the heels and other dry areas. Look for products that contain ingredients like urea, glycerin, or lactic acid, which can help to soften and hydrate the skin.

- Trim your toenails regularly and straight across to prevent ingrown toenails.

- Wear clean socks made of breathable materials, such as cotton or bamboo, and change them daily. Avoid wearing socks that are too tight or restrictive, as this can cause rubbing and irritation.

- Choose shoes that fit well and provide adequate support. Avoid high heels or shoes with narrow, pointed toes, as these can put pressure on the heels and toes.

- Give your feet a break throughout the day by taking frequent breaks to stretch and walk around, especially if you have a job that requires standing or sitting for long periods of time.

- Protect your feet from injury by wearing shoes or sandals in public places like pools and locker rooms, and avoid going barefoot outside.

Proper Footwear:

Choose shoes that fit properly and provide adequate support. Avoid wearing shoes that are too tight or too loose, as these can cause rubbing and pressure on the heels. Consider wearing shoes with a wider toe box and cushioned soles to reduce pressure on the heels.

- Choose shoes that fit well: Shoes that are too tight or too loose can put pressure on your heels, causing them to crack. Make sure your shoes fit properly and provide enough support for your feet.

- Avoid high heels: High heels can put a lot of pressure on your heels and cause them to crack. If you must wear heels, choose shoes with a lower heel and wear them for shorter periods of time.

- Wear socks: Socks can help keep your feet moisturized and prevent dry skin. Look for socks made from natural fibers, such as cotton or wool, which allow your feet to breathe.

- Use insoles or orthotics: Insoles or orthotics can help provide extra cushioning and support for your feet, reducing the risk of cracked heels.

- Avoid open-back shoes: Shoes that are open at the back, such as sandals or flip-flops, can cause your heels to dry out and crack. If you must wear open-back shoes, choose ones with a supportive sole and wear them for shorter periods of time.

Hydration:

- Drink plenty of water to keep your skin hydrated from the inside out. Aim for at least 8 glasses of water per day.
- Drink plenty of water throughout the day to stay hydrated from the inside out.
- Apply a moisturizing cream or lotion to your feet daily, especially after bathing or showering when the skin is most absorbent.
- Soak your feet in warm water for 10-15 minutes before applying a moisturizing cream or lotion. This can help to soften the skin and make it more receptive to the moisturizer.
- Avoid hot water when bathing or showering, as this can strip the skin of natural oils and lead to dryness.
- Wear socks made from breathable materials, such as cotton or wool, to help keep your feet dry and reduce the risk of developing fungal infections.

Balanced Diet: Eating a balanced diet that is rich in vitamins and minerals can help keep your skin healthy and prevent dryness. Incorporate foods that are high in vitamin A and E, such as sweet potatoes, carrots, almonds, and spinach.

Maintaining a balanced diet is important for overall health, including foot health. Certain nutrients can help promote healthy skin and prevent dryness, which can contribute to cracked heels. These include:

- Omega-3 fatty acids: Found in fish, nuts, and seeds, omega-3 fatty acids can help reduce inflammation and improve skin health.

- Vitamin E: Found in nuts, seeds, and leafy green vegetables, vitamin E is an antioxidant that can help protect the skin and prevent dryness.

- Vitamin C: Found in citrus fruits, berries, and leafy green vegetables, vitamin C is essential for collagen production, which is important for skin health.

- Zinc: Found in meat, seafood, and legumes, zinc is important for skin healing and can help prevent infections.

- Water: Staying hydrated by drinking plenty of water can help prevent dry skin and promote overall foot health.

Foot Soaks:

Soaking your feet in warm water can help to soften and moisturize dry skin. Consider adding Epsom salts or essential oils, such as lavender or tea tree oil, to the water for added benefits.

Foot soaks can be a relaxing and effective way to help soothe and soften dry, cracked heels. Some common ingredients used in foot soaks include:

- Epsom salt: Epsom salt is a popular ingredient in foot soaks due to its high magnesium content, which can help to relax muscles and soothe soreness. It can also help to soften and exfoliate the skin.

- Apple cider vinegar: Apple cider vinegar has antimicrobial properties that can help to fight off infections and fungus. It can also help to balance the pH of the skin and reduce inflammation.

- Baking soda: Baking soda can help to exfoliate and soften the skin, and its alkaline properties can help to balance the pH of the skin.

- Essential oils: Essential oils such as lavender, tea tree, and peppermint can be added to foot soaks for their soothing and antimicrobial properties.

Avoid Harsh Soaps: Avoid using harsh soaps or detergents on your feet, as these can strip the skin of its natural oils and contribute to dryness.

Harsh soaps can strip the skin of its natural oils and contribute to dryness, which can lead to cracked heels. It is recommended to use mild, fragrance-free soaps to avoid further irritation and dryness. Additionally, it is important to rinse the feet thoroughly after washing to ensure that all soap residue is removed.

Regular Exfoliation: Regularly exfoliating your feet with a pumice stone or foot file can help to remove dead skin cells and prevent buildup, which can contribute to cracking.

Regular exfoliation of the feet can help to remove dead skin cells and prevent the buildup of thick, dry skin that can contribute to cracked heels. There are several methods of exfoliation that can be used, including:

- Pumice stone: A pumice stone is a natural stone made from volcanic rock that can be used to gently scrub away dead skin cells from the feet.

- Foot scrub: A foot scrub is a product that contains small particles, such as sugar or salt, that can be used to exfoliate the feet. Simply apply the scrub to the feet and massage in a circular motion before rinsing off.

- Foot file: A foot file is a tool that can be used to file away rough, dry skin on the feet. Use a gentle back-and-forth motion to avoid causing any damage to the skin.

Prevention from foot cracks includes:

- Keeping the feet well-moisturized with a good foot cream or lotion.

- Wearing comfortable, well-fitted shoes that do not put excessive pressure on the heels or toes.

- Avoiding harsh soaps and detergents that can strip the skin of its natural oils.

- Maintaining good hygiene by regularly washing and drying the feet.

- Exfoliating the feet regularly to remove dead skin cells and prevent the buildup of calluses.

- Eating a balanced diet rich in vitamins and minerals that are important for skin health.

- Staying hydrated by drinking plenty of water throughout the day.

- Avoiding prolonged exposure to hot water or harsh chemicals, which can dry out the skin.

- Treating any underlying medical conditions, such as diabetes or psoriasis, that may increase the risk of developing cracked heels.
- Seeking medical treatment if home remedies are not effective or if the cracks become infected or painful.

By incorporating these tips into your daily routine, you can help to maintain healthy feet and prevent future episodes of cracked heels.

Conclusion:

In conclusion, cracked heels, also known as heel fissures, are a common foot problem that can cause discomfort and even pain. Proper foot care can help prevent and repair cracked heels. Here are some tips to help repair cracked heels:

- Soak your feet in warm water for 10-15 minutes to help soften the skin, and then gently exfoliate the dry, thickened skin with a pumice stone.

- Apply a thick layer of moisturizing cream or lotion to the affected areas, focusing on the heels. Petroleum jelly or other emollients can also be used.

- Cover the moisturizer with a pair of socks to help the skin absorb the cream and to prevent further drying.

- Wear comfortable, well-fitting shoes that provide good support and cushioning for your feet.

- Avoid wearing open-back shoes, as they can cause the skin to become dry and cracked.

- If you have severe cracking, apply a moisturizing cream containing urea or lactic acid, which can help soften and break down the thickened skin.

- If your cracked heels are accompanied by pain, bleeding, or signs of infection, seek medical attention.

By following these tips and incorporating good foot care practices into your daily routine, you can help prevent and repair cracked heels and maintain healthy, pain-free feet.

Your review means

a lot to me...

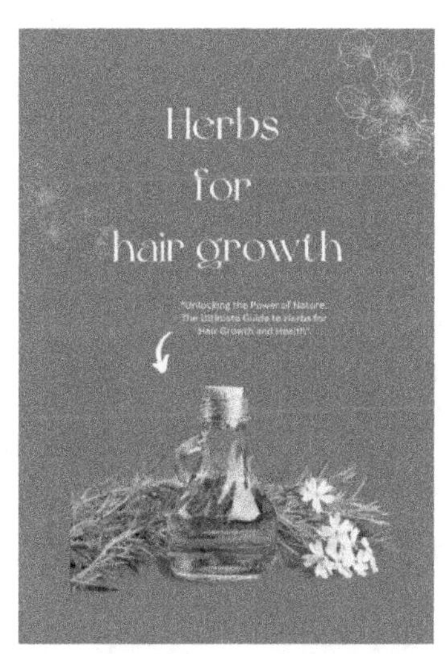

Herbs
for
hair growth
Unlocking the Power of Nature:
The Ultimate Guide to Herbs for
Hair Growth and Health

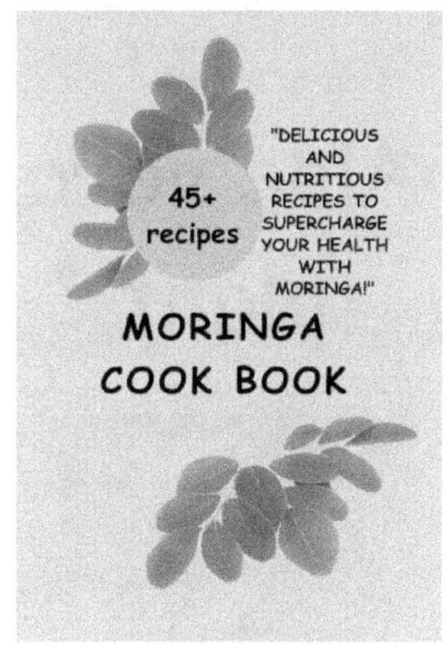

45+
recipes
"DELICIOUS
AND
NUTRITIOUS
RECIPES TO
SUPERCHARGE
YOUR HEALTH
WITH
MORINGA!"
MORINGA
COOK BOOK

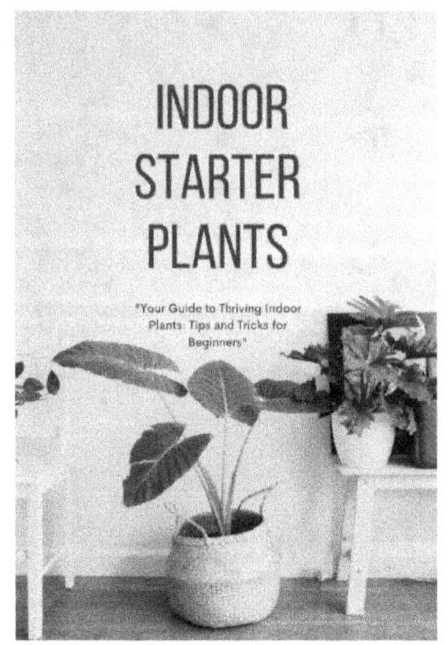

Aloe vera plant

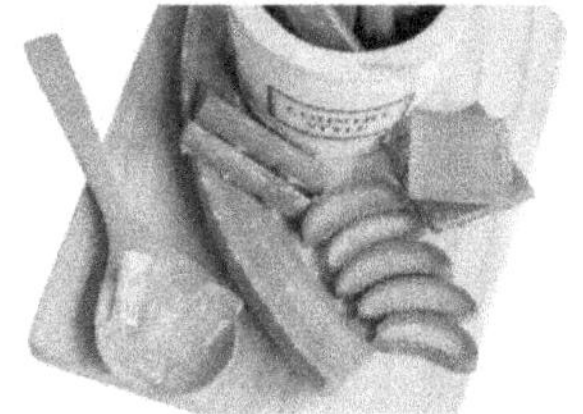

herbal remedies